Poems for Children

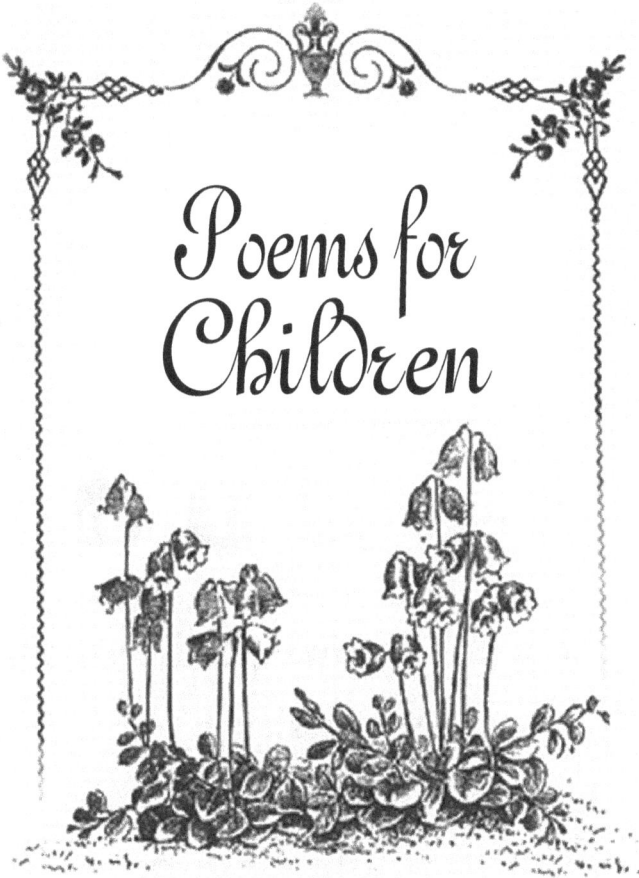

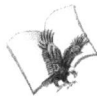

V&S PUBLISHERS

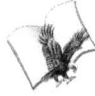

Published by:

$\mathcal{V}\&S$ PUBLISHERS

F-2/16, Ansari Road, Daryaganj, New Delhi-110002
011-23240026, 011-23240027 • *Fax:* 011-23240028
Email: info@vspublishers.com • *Website:* www.vspublishers.com

Branch : Hyderabad
5-1-707/1, Brij Bhawan (Beside Central Bank of India Lane)
Bank Street, Koti, Hyderabad - 500 095
040-24737290
E-mail: vspublishershyd@gmail.com

Follow us on:

For any assistance sms **VSPUB** to **56161**

All books available at **www.vspublishers.com**

© **Copyright:** $\mathcal{V}\&S$ PUBLISHERS
ISBN 978-93-505705-1-7
Edition 2013

Printed at : Param Offseters, Okhla, New Delhi-110020

PREFACE

A small poem consists of the inner feelings of a person condensed in verse. It displays innocence and sweetness, when written by a school-going child. Children express their thoughts, emotions, likes, dislikes and other innermost feelings in a free and frank manner. Most of the small poems compiled in this book are written by schoolchildren, besides some by famous poets. I have made a few small changes and have also included a few poems of my own. When small children express their thoughts and feelings in verse, these come straight from their hearts. They try to say what they actually feel inside without any fear or favour. The poems included in this book cover a wide variety of subjects which encompass feelings of love for their parents, teachers, companions, country and expression of interest in things which they come across amidst their childhood and school environment. Coming from the hearts and minds of innocent children, these poems will no doubt provide a spontaneous source of delight, amusement, information, education and general pleasure.

I am confident that this compilation of sweet and educative poems will be welcomed by students, their teachers and parents besides the general readers.

Since, it is a collective effort by the school students, some of the poems maybe a little sarcastic or humorous in nature, but they are all intended for fun and should be taken lightly by our esteemed readers.

CONTENTS

SMILE – COME WHAT MAY

Smile, come what may
It keeps problems at bay
A smiling face is bright sunshine
It keeps you fit happy and fine
When something troubles you must smile
Will keep it away at least for a while
A smile brings a glimmer of ray
And makes your day a happy day
And happy days
Will make a pile
When you smile, smile and more smile.

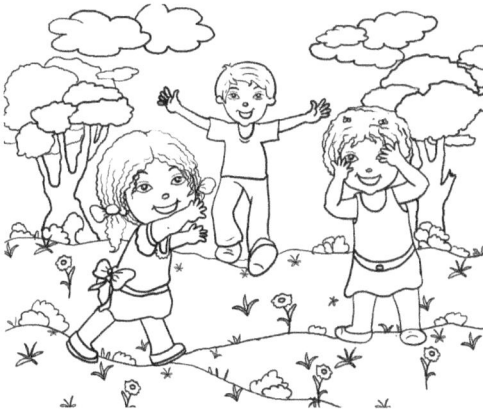

WHO MOST LIVES

One most lives
Who thinks most
Feels the noblest,
And acts the best.

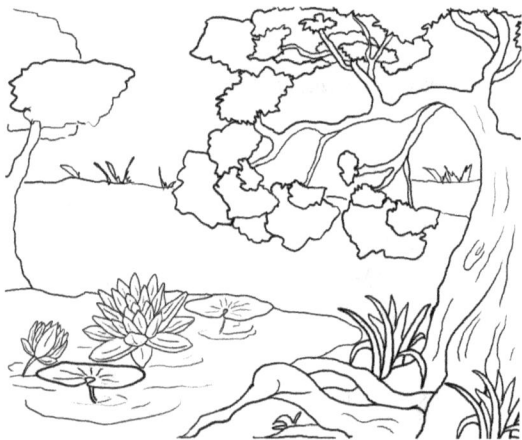

DEAR PARENTS

You are like a prayer
To me.
Without your love and care
Life seems to me
Searching for a cover.
How can I even think
Of losing my way
When you are guiding me
To move and stay
You are the breath
I take
And the thoughts
I think
You are my everything
I truly need your blessing.
And nothing compares
With you
My life is all yours
And all my dreams
Belong to you.

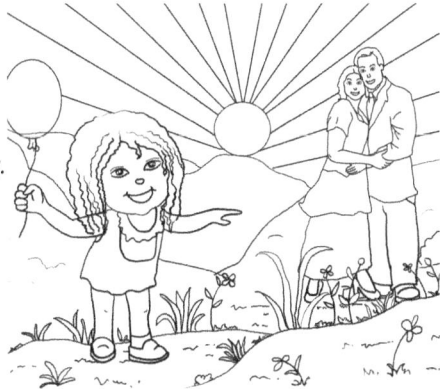

DO NOT FIND FAULT

There is so much good in worst of us
And so much bad in the best of us
That it will not behave and one of us
To find any fault with the rest of us.
(R.L. STEVENSON)

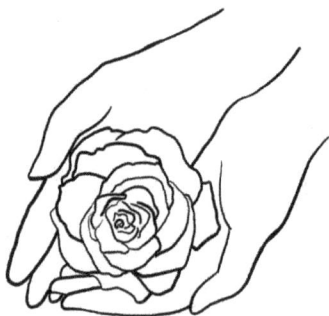

THE DAYS GO BY

We live and work and dream
Each has his little scheme
Sometimes we cry
And thus the days go by!

GREED

The world is enough for everyone's needs
But not ever enough for one man's greed!

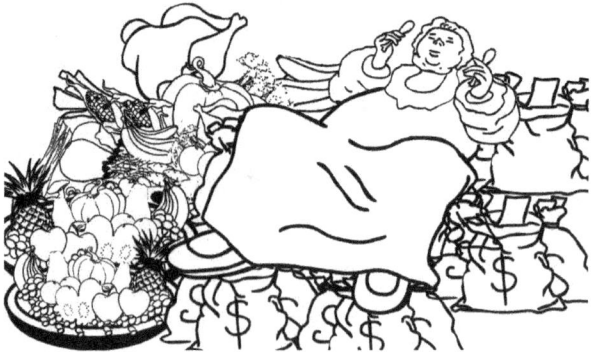

PRESENT TIME

For yesterday is but a dream
And tomorrow only a vision
But today well lived, makes every yesterday
A dream of happiness
And every tomorrow
A vision of hope and joy
Look well then to this day.
(KAVI KALIDAS)

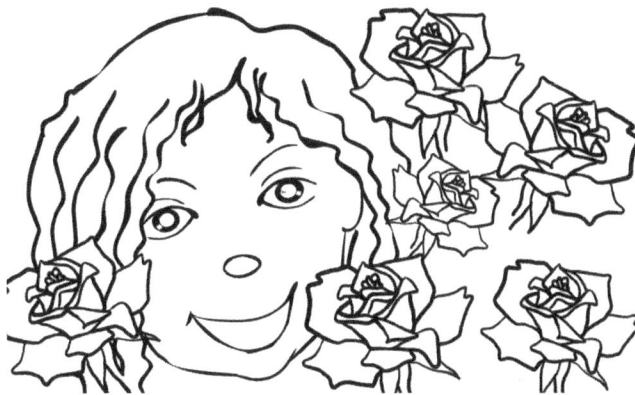

HABITS, GOOD AND BAD

Good habits are difficult to acquire
But easy to live with.
Bad habits are easy to acquire
But difficult to live with.

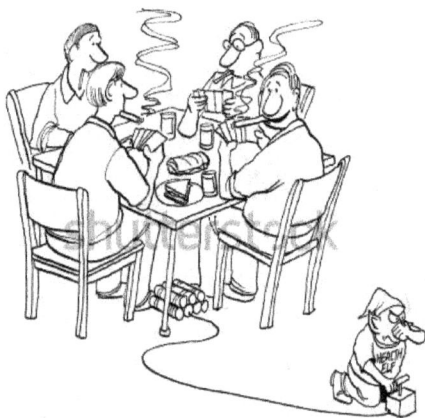

CHANGE

Life always changes
Time always changes
Money always changes
Man always changes
Age decreases, desire increases
Change is the law of nature
So into fit your status!

INVEST FOR THE BETTER WORLD

If you want to exist
In a world better
Then you have to invest
In its future which is a child
So give him good case and guide
Invest in him with full pride
For a better world.

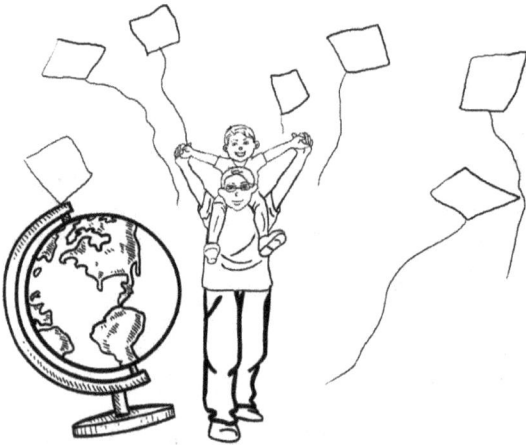

LOVE, WORK AND LAUGH

Love and leave anger
Work and leave hunger
Laugh and live longer
And make your life stronger.

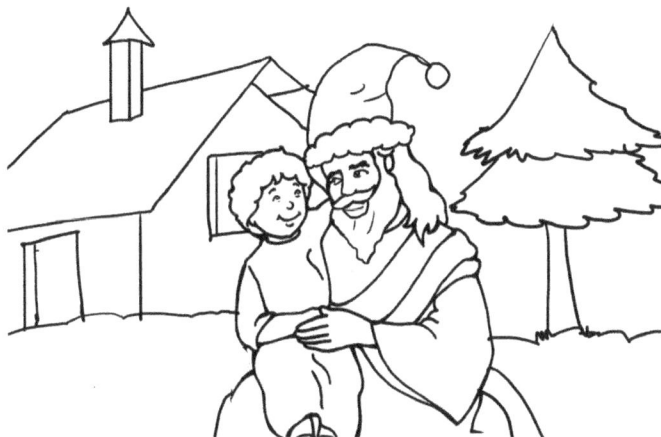

GREAT LOSS

Where is the life?
We have lost in living!
Where is the wisdom?
We have lost in knowledge!
Where is the knowledge?
We have lost in information!
So life has been a great loss
What should we do about it?

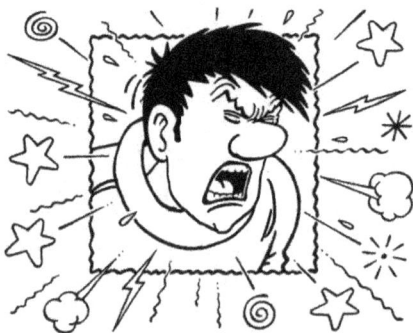

RECIPE FOR A HAPPY DAY

Take one pound of sheer kindness
And stir it well
With good thoughts that bless
Add plenty of patience to make it nice
Some good fun will add a little spice
Do not weigh love, just pour it anyway
Mix it well, you will make it a happy day.

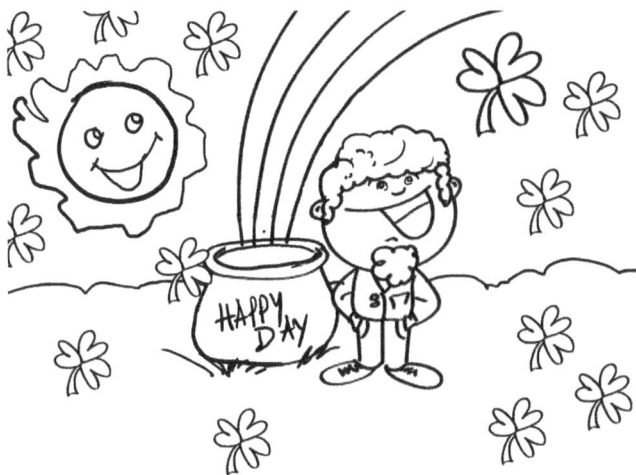

LIFE AND DEATH

Each day is a little life
Waking and rising and all strife
Which make active a little youth
And every rest and sleep a little death!

USE OF TIME

Of the twenty-four hours of a day
Use six for earning and spending pay
Six for thought of God and pray
Six for sleep and six for service and play.

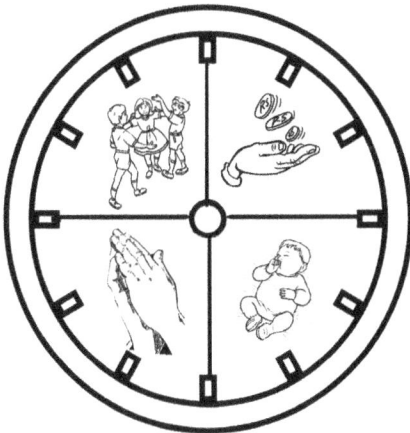

FRUITS OF EVIL DEEDS

Neither in the sky
Nor on mountain high
Nor in deepest caves
Where ocean water raves
Nor anywhere on earth indeed
Where men and women can escape
The fruits of their evil deeds.

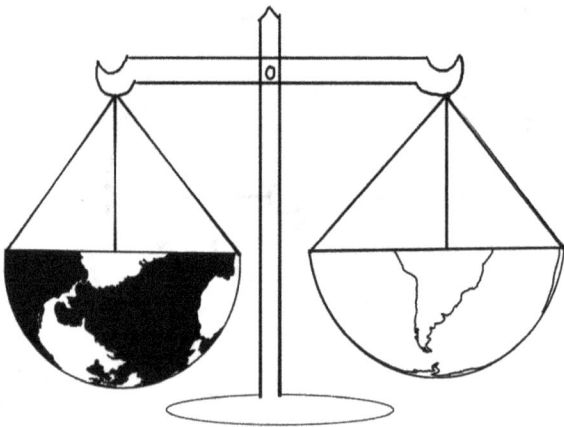

TIME

Time flies, airmen say
Time marches, soldiers say
Time and tide
Wait for none, sailors say
Let us use our time
For our good and that of fellow men.

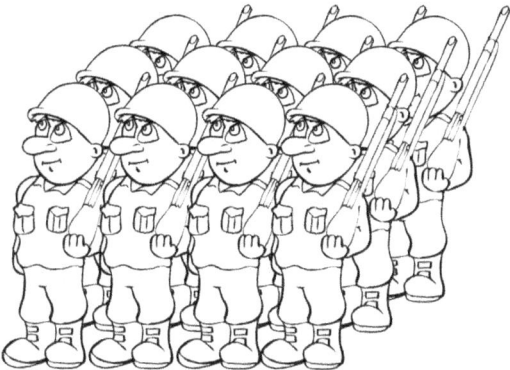

SPEAK GENTLY

Speak gently; it is better far
To rule by love than fear
Speak gently; lest a harsh word mar
The good we may do here
Speak gently; to the little child
Its love be sure to gain
Teach it in accents soft and mild
It may not long remain
Speak gently, to the aged one
Grieve not the care worn heart
Where sounds of life are nearly run
Let such in peace depart
Speak gently; it is a little thing
Dropped in the heart's deep well
The good the joy that it may bring
Eternally shall I'll...

(H.W. LONG FELLOW)

SMILE

Smile with others
And share your joy
Smile at your wife
And remove all strife
Smile at your mate
To cheer his life
Smile at your kids
And make them friends
Smile at all and every one
And always be kind
Give your gentle love
And leave hatred behind.

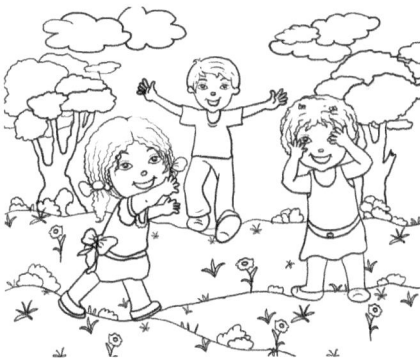

WHAT A LIFE!

What is life
It's full of care
And we have no time
To stand and stare!

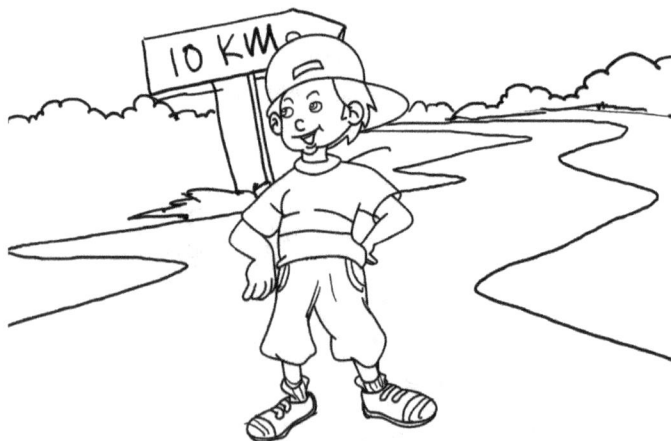

SWEET LITTLE CHILD

How sweet and pleasant
Is the face of an infant?
He is sheer joy
God and nature's toy
His smile so pure
An instant cure
Which brings gladness
And remove all sadness
A sweet little angel
He knows no evil
How tiny sweet and small
He is loved by one and all.

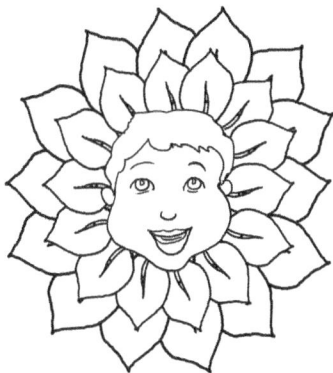

NEVER TROUBLE

Better never trouble, trouble
Until trouble, troubles you
For you only make you trouble
Double trouble when you do!

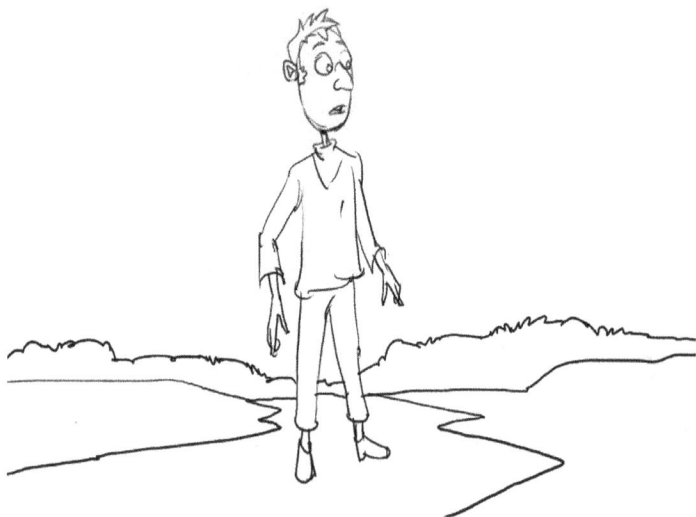

MOTHER IS SPECIAL

She gave us birth
Made our life full of worth
For us she takes so much pain
And saves us from sun and rain
She teaches us good manners
And to speak truth without a stammer
She lends us dignity
And leads us to our destiny
She guides us with grace
And makes our world a better place
There is no one who can take her place
Since God cannot be seen everywhere
So He created something special, a Mother!

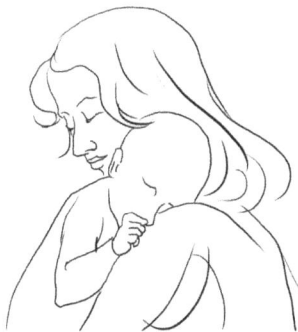

GREAT MEN

Lives of great men
All remind us
We can make our lives sublime
And departing
Leave behind us
Footprints on the sands of time
(H.W. LONGFELLOW)

SWEET MOTHER

Breathes there a sound
Above all others
Sweetest in the world
To me
It is the sacred name
Of mother
Which is very clear
To me
I do not know of
All the sorrows
For me she gladly bore
But I do know this
With every tomorrow
In her heart
She loved me more and more
Oh sweet mother
I see God in her!

TIME IS ALWAYS MOVING

Time has no beginning
It has no end.
It is always running
And never bends.

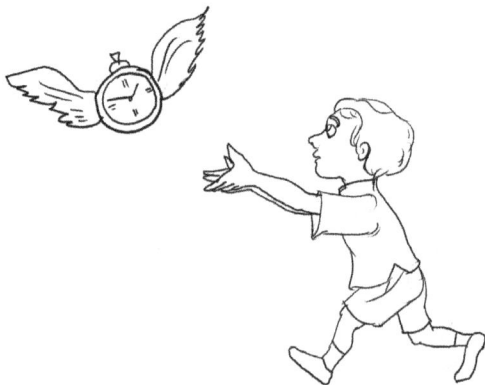

TIME WAITS FOR NONE

Time and tide
Never lag behind
That is why
The wise cry
These wait for none
So well begun
Is half done.

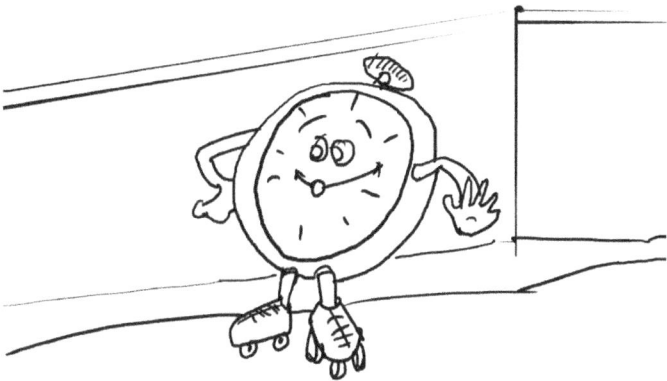

TIME MATTERS

Time in all ages
Has three stages
First is the past
That is already lost
Second is the present
Which is still current
Third is the future
Which has no stature
Since past is dead
Do not know its end
And nobody knows
How future grows
But soon it rolls
Into the present's fold
So it is the present
Which really matters
So make it pleasant
And make it better.

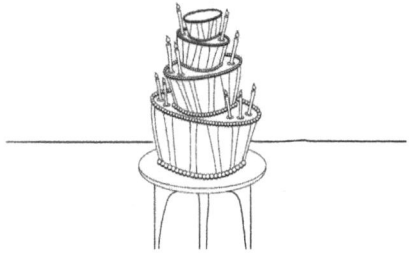

LET US ALWAYS LEARN

Learn from the ants
To work very hard
Learn from the flowers
To be very kind
Learn from the mountains
To be very strong
Learn from the rivers
To be always firm
Learn from the birds
To fly in the air
Learn from the bees
To always keep busy.

NOBEL THOUGHTS

Let your aims be common
And your hearts of one accord
And all of you be of one mind
So that you may live well together!
                    (FROM RIGVEDA)

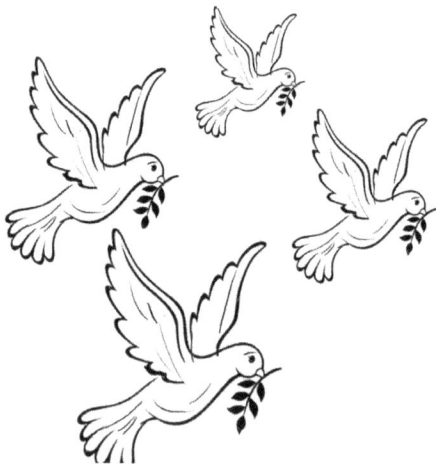

HELP OTHERS

HELP, as much as you can
As lovingly, as you can
As efficiently, as you can
Do not leave for result
But thank God with respect
That He gave you
A chance to serve others.

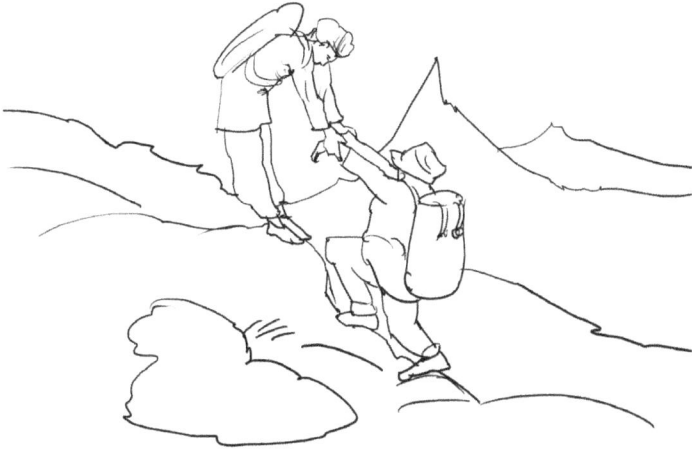

GOD WILL ASK YOU

Tomorrow or later
God is not going to ask
What did you dream?
Or did you eat cream?
What did you think?
Or did your eyes blink?
What did you plan?
Or which is your clan?
What did you preach?
Or what was within reach?
But he is certainly going to ask
What did you do?

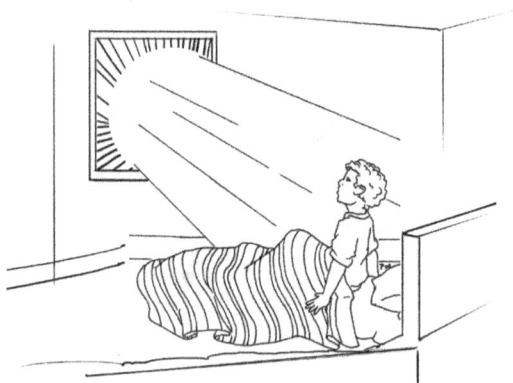

GOD KEEPS THE KEY

Life is a story
In volumes three
The past the present and
The yet to be
The first is finished
And laid away
The second we are reading
Day by day
The third and last of
The volumes three
Is locked from sight and
God keeps the key!

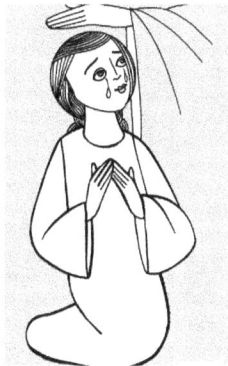

YOU WILL DO IT

There may be thousands
To tell you
It cannot be done
There may be thousands
To say to you
The dangers that wait to assail you
But you just tackle in
With a bit of grin
And get in
Just start to sing
As you tackle the thing
Which others said
It cannot be done
But you will do it.

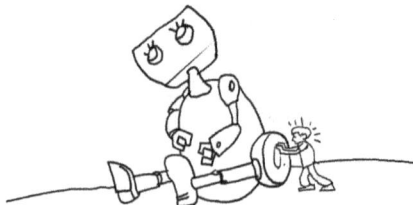

THE CHILD

Child a little lord
Is capable of becoming GOD
Every childbirth is a victory
Every new born is a prophecy
To be a prophet
One must remain a child
Children take their play seriously
Men make their life tragically
The nearer a man is to God
The more he feels himself a child.

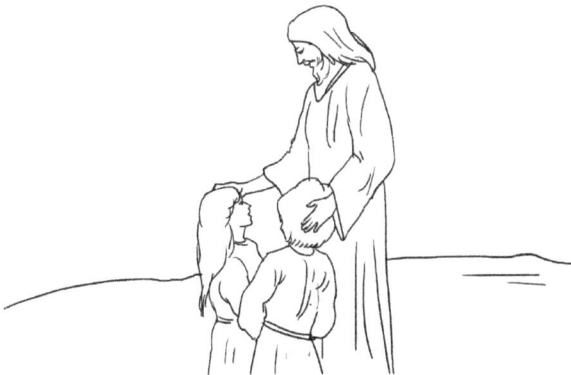

TEACHERS

Teachers are so bright
Full of confidence and light
They show us the path of life
And make us wise and nice
Sometime they guide us with a stick
But also love and help when we are sick
I love my teachers much
They are like preachers as such.

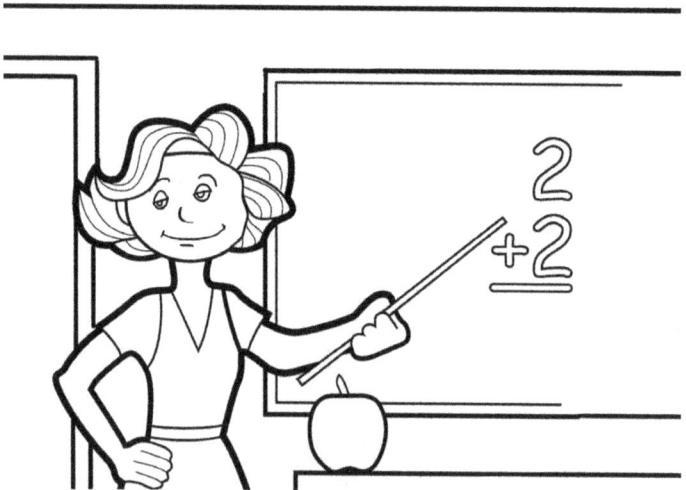

BE A LEADER

The boss drives his men
The leader inspires them
The boss demands skills
The leader wants goodwill
The boss evokes fear
The leader wipes tears
The boss says 'I'
The leader says 'WE'
The boss shows who is wrong
The leader says what is wrong
The boss knows how it is done
The leader shows how to do it
The boss abuses man
The leader uses them
The boss demands respect
The leader commands respect.

(ANONYMOUS)

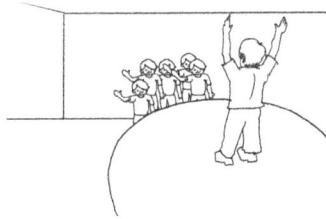

BEWARE

Beware of the man
No says he can
But does not do it
Beware of the man
Who says all is mine
And everything is fine
Beware of the man
Who says nothing is good
And all fault is there
Beware of the man
Who cannot scan
What is good or bad?
And makes you sad!

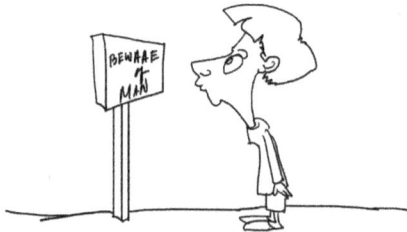

HEALTH vs WEALTH

Then lose their health
For getting wealthy
Then lose their wealth
For getting healthy
Better keep your health
Do not run after wealth.

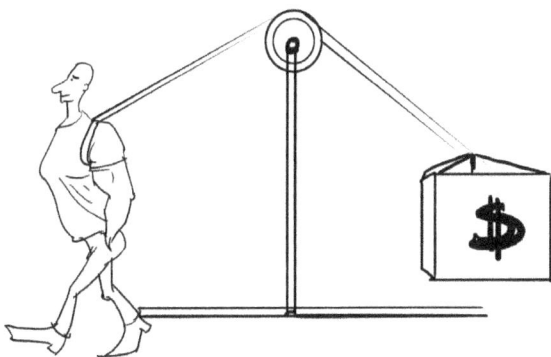

OUR ACTS

Act repeated
Leads to a habit
Every habit
Behaviour directs
And all behaviour
Character makes
From the character
Our life takes
Its sorrows and joys
And keeps on playing
With these toys.

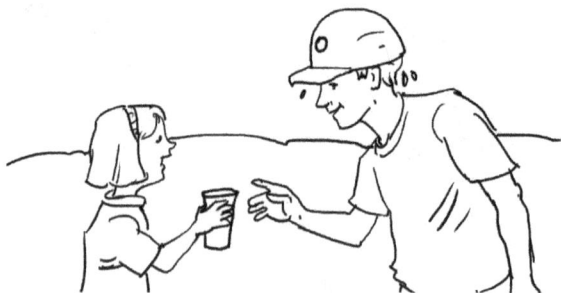

LOVE NOT HATE

We are born to love
Not to hate
We are born to work
Not to wait on fate
Make it a habit
Never to be late
If you do so
Success is at your gate.

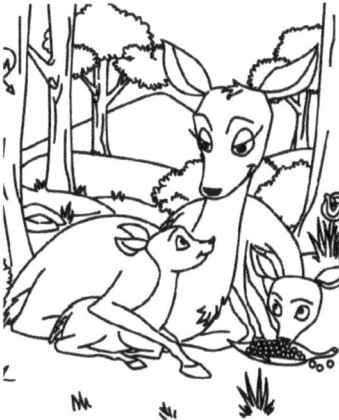

SMILE IS A TREASURE

A smile is a treasure
Which you cannot measure
Smile and the world
Will smile with you
And when you cry
You will cry alone
So have no fear
And wipe your tears
Forget your sadness
And let a sweet smile
Bring you gladness.

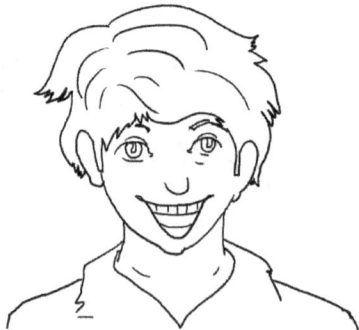

A FRIEND INDEED

A friend in need
Is a friend indeed
Fathers indeed are
Those who feed
True comrades are wives indeed
When trust and sweet contents proceed.

JOY AND SORROW

Joy and sorrow
Whether today or tomorrow
None other brings to us
Our own deeds (word missing page no 24)
These are our own fruit
In every pursuit
Therefore we need not complain
With any distain
Some other beings
For our own doings!

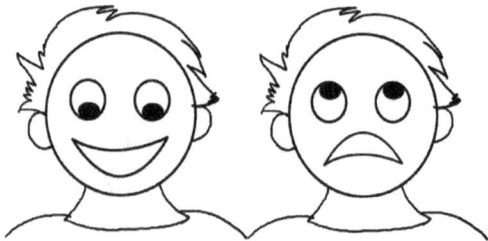

ARITHMETIC OF LIFE

May our life be arithmetic
Our grief be subtracted
And sorrows divided
Let joys be added
And happiness multiplied.

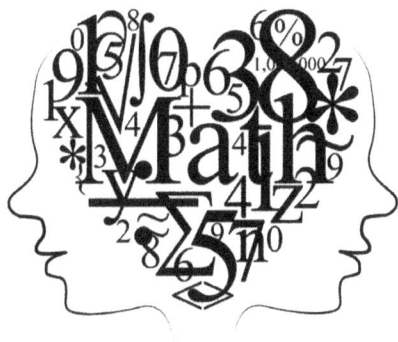

THE MAKING Of A MOTHER

God took the fragrance
Of a flower
The majesty of a tree
The calm of a quiet sea
The gentlemen of morning hour
The beauty of twilight hours
The soul of a starry night
The grace of a bird in flight
An angel's tender care
The laughter of a jumping river
The patience of eternity
Its depth and serenity
From all these he fashioned
A living creature
A masterpiece like now other
But he called it simply a MOTHER.

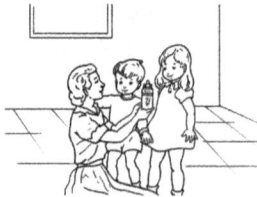

MY LOVE FOR INDIA

Roses may weep
And thorns may cry
But my love for INDIA
Will never die
Get up go, join the race
Don't feel tired
And keep the pace
Poverty, hunger, hatred of caste
I wish GANDHIJI came from the past
qNever, never
Oh never give up
We all will join
And help you rise high and up.

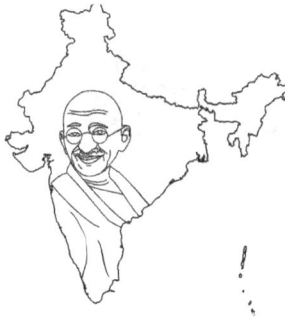

WEAR A SMILE

One is not completely dressed
Unless one wears a smile.

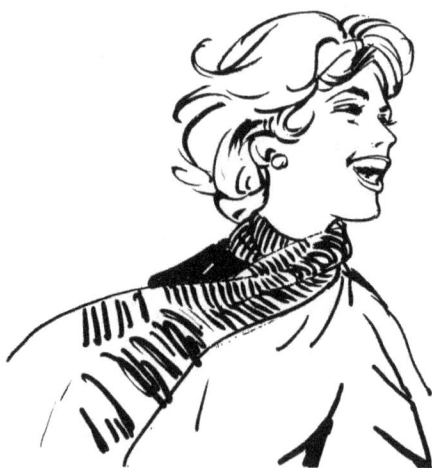

ONLY ONE MOTHER

Hundreds of stars in the dark sky
Hundreds of birds who sing and fly
Hundreds of shells on the seaside
Hundreds of bees in the golden hive
Hundreds of dew drops to greet the dawn
Hundreds of butterflies in the lawn
But there is only one MOTHER
The whole wide world over!

FRIENDS AND FOES

Some friends appear foes
Some foes appear friends
To gain their own ends
Never put your trust
In evil friends
Foolish false with selfish ends!

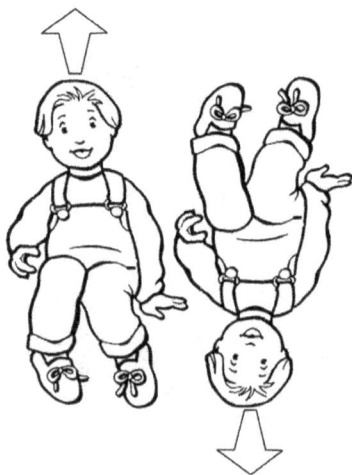

THE WORLD – A FAMILY

The world is a family
To live in harmony
Working all the while
Sharing with a smile
This knowledge we must treasure
And use it to help our earth
Let us boys and girls all over the world
Unite, work and show our worth.

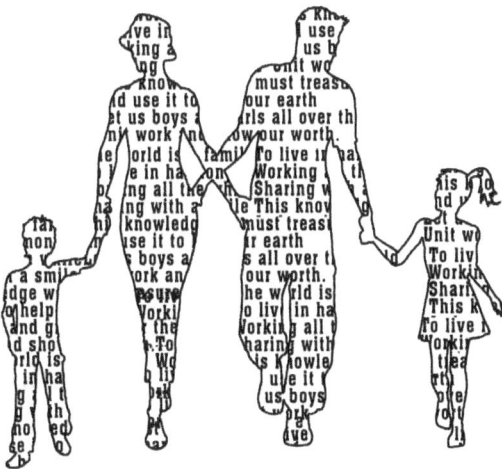

THE MESSAGE OF MARRIAGE

When you marry someone, love him
After your marriage, study him
If he is honest, respect him
If he is generous, appreciate him
When he is sad, cheer him
When he is glad, share with him
If he is in some trouble, bear with him
If he is noble, praise him
If he is social, encourage him
If he is jealous, cure him
But always try to trust him.

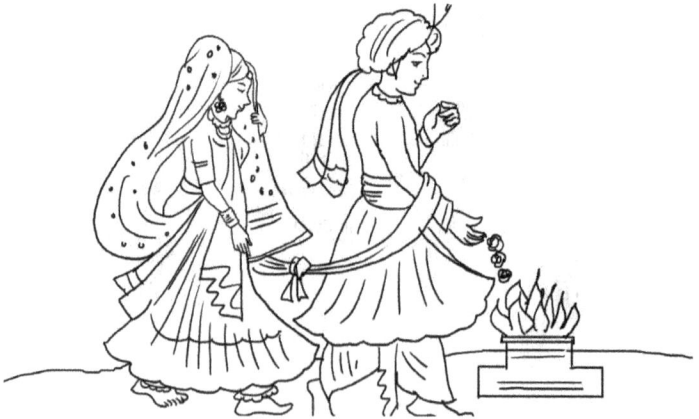

AIM OF MY LIFE

The aim of my life
Is very noble and nice
My aim is to become a surgeon
To help the needy poor persons
I will cure diseases of patients
By doing difficult operations
In surgery, I will set new trends
Surgical instruments will be my friends
I know this is a difficult aim
It needs hard work and pain
To serve God and the mankind
This motto will be on my mind
God give me strength to achieve my aim
With your help, success I will claim.

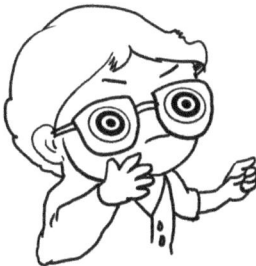

LEARN TO LABOUR AND TO WAIT

Tell me not in mournful numbers
Life is but, an empty dream!
For the soul is dead that
Slumbers
And things are not what they
Seem
Life is real! Life is earnest!
And the grave is not its goal
Dust than art to dust returnest
Was not spoken of the soul
Let us make up and doing
With a heart for any fate
Still achieving, still pursuing
Learn to labour, and to wait
(H.W. LONGFELLOW)

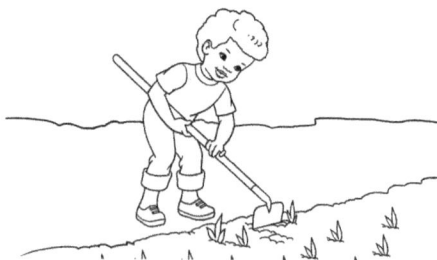

ONE MORE TRY

It is easy to cry that you are
Beaten and die
It is easy to crawfish
And crawl
But to fight and to fight
When hope's out of sight
Why that's the best
Game of all
And though you come out of
Each gruelling bout
All broken and beaten
And scarred
Just have one more try
It's dead easy to die
It is the keeping on
Living that is hard.

THE APPROPRIATE TIME

A disciple of Lord BUDDHA saw a beggar on the road and started giving sermon to him. But the beggar was in no mood to listen to the preacher even though the latter made his best efforts. Finally when the preacher got disgusted he went back to BUDDHA and expressed his disappointment. Lord BUDDHA smiled and said, "Ok, you bring him I will teach him personally. The disciple brought the beggar and Buddha asked another disciple to take him to the kitchen and make him eat his fill. The first disciple was annoyed and asked the Lord, "But you have not given him any sermon!"

Buddha smiled again and said, "Today he needs food. I will give him sermon tomorrow."

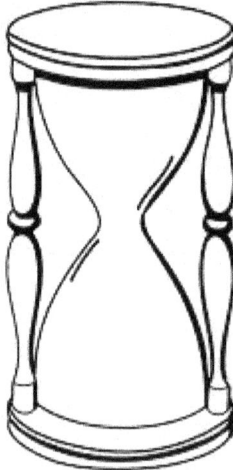

A DIALOGUE WITH GOD

God told man
To build a better world
And man questioned, 'How'?
The world is large
And I am small
There is not much, I can do!
But GOD, all wise and kind
Smiled and said
Just Build A BETTER You.

MAKER OF A HOUSE

The beauty of a home
Is in harmony
The security of a home
Is in loyalty
The pleasure of a house
Is in kids
The rule of a house
Is in love
But the real maker of a home
Is GOD HIMSELF.

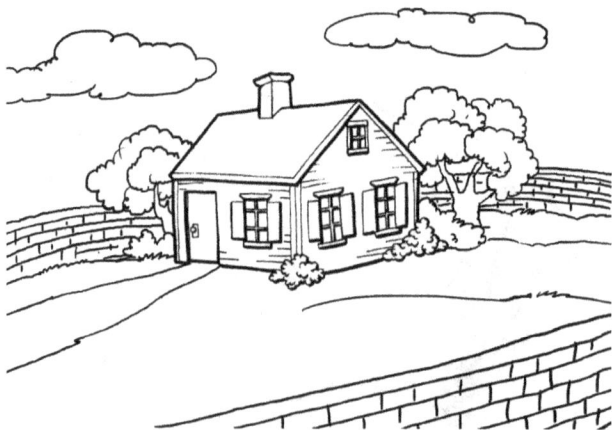

OUR BRAVE WARRIORS

Your spirit is mightier
Than the mountain ranges
Your aim is holier
Than the holy ganges
You are faster
Than rain and air
Your strength makes
Your enemy scare
When you speak
Through your gun
The Enemy is bound to run
We in the present
Are lucky to see you
And those in the future
Are keenly waiting for you
Oh brave soldiers, we all salute you!

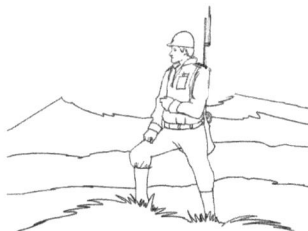

TIME AND PLACE FOR EVERYTHING

There is time and place
For everything
And a mind which governs
Them all
There is hidden doubt
In a wish
And comfort in a fall
But how not your head
To life's furious hammer
Rather break the shackle that binds
And at destiny's gate clamours'
For when all is said and done
You are young and free
And though dreams may
Appear distant
You are today all
You ever need to be.

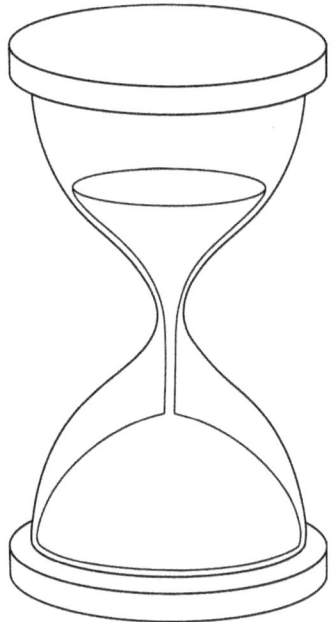

A VERY INTERESTING LETTER (READ IT LIKE A POEM)

(THE OTHER VERSION OF EARLIER LETTER)

The more I think of you, the more I hate you: you have always been to me an object of contempt.
It is true that once I said I loved you. That assertion you know was a lie and I do not know why I made it. If I offer you my hand and know very well you would accept it. I do not think I would make my whole life miserable. To die would be preferable to that if you write to me I shall be miserable and gloomy, your letter always make me feel like committing sucide.

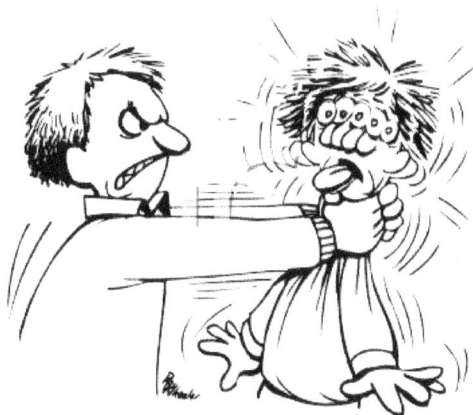

ALPHABET FOR SUCCESS

A. Should keep you ACTIVE

B. Inspires you to be BOLD

C. Makes you a good CITIZEN

D. Keeps you DUTIFUL

E. Asks you to respect ELDERS

F. Tells you to be FAITHFUL

G. Makes you GENTLE

H. Advises you to be HONEST

I. Expects you to be INTELLIGENT

J. Teaches you to be JUST

K. Asks you to be KIND

L. Wishes you to be LOVING

M. Asks you to be MERCIFUL

N. Makes you NEAT

O. Makes you OBEDIENT

P. Asks you to be PUNCTUAL

Q. Says keep QUIET

R. Teaches you to be REGULAR

S. Stands for SERVICE

T. Tells you to be TRUTHFUL

U. Warns about the UNEXPECTED

V. Cultivates VIRTUE

W. Be wealthy and WISE

X. Stands for EXCELLENCE

Y. Inspires YOUTH

Z. Is for Zeal.

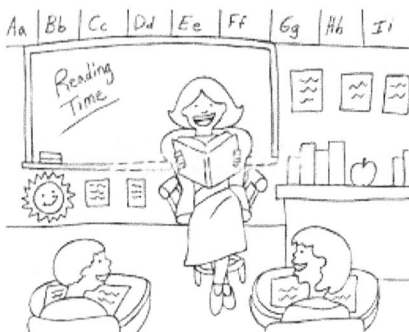

WAKE UP WOMEN!

Wake up women please do not sleep

And show the your real zeal

You can be SITA

And also MOTHER TERESA

And the RANI OF JHANSI

To fight the FIRANGIES

Wake up and show your power

Tell the world what you can shower!

Fight for justice and fight for truth

And never fear in old age or youth

Wake up women wake up

March forward and shake up!

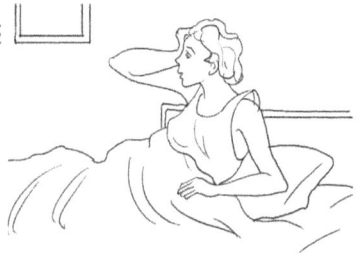

FAILURE

Failure is when you lose the hope

Failure is when you cry and grope

Failure is one who weeps and shelters

Failure is one who blames and betters

Failure is one who gets depressed

Failure is one whom ignorance pressed

So be bold and never fail

Keep running like a rail.

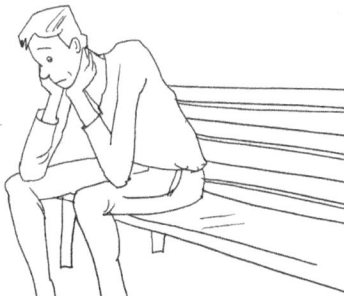

TWINKLE, TWINKLE

Twinkle, twinkle little star,

How I wonder what you are?

Up above the world so high,

Like a diamond in the sky.

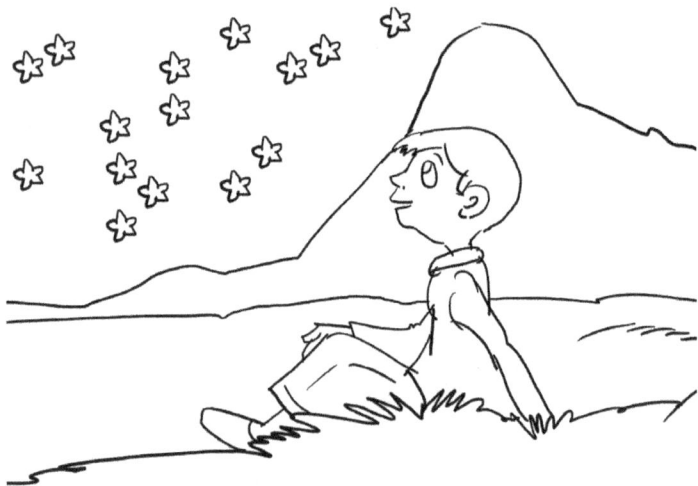

FROM RIGVEDA

Let your aims be common

And your hearts of our accord

And all of you be one mind

So that you may live well together.

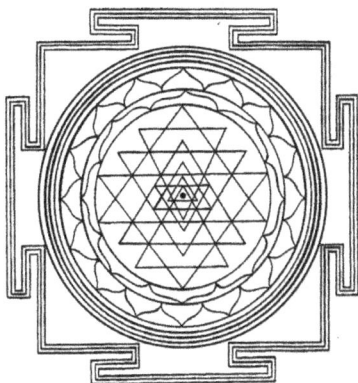

FROM SRI GURU GRANTH SAHIB

Greed is a dark prison house

The sins committed out of greed

Become fetters round one's feet.

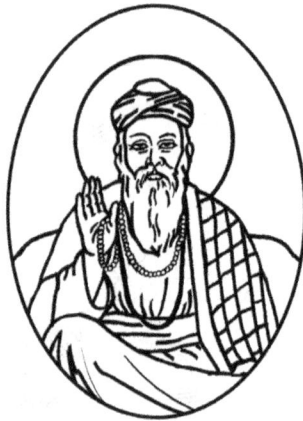

SRI AUROBINDO

However dark the night

We cannot lose faith in the dawn

The darkest nights prepare the brightest dawns

So, we must not despair and give up.

SHELLEY

If winter comes

Can spring be far behind?

SIX HONEST SERVING MEN

I keep six honest serving men

Their names are what, why and when

How, where and WHO?

(RUDYARD KIPLING)

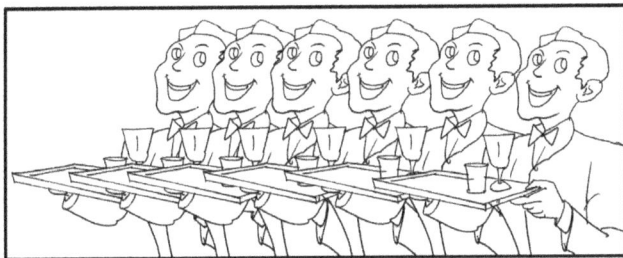

THE ROOT OF ALL EVIL

Money is the root of all evil

And its greed that makes a man a devil

Man loves money

As a bee loves honey

Man wants to amass wealth

Without caring for his health

When hoarding wealth becomes prime

It can lead to many a crime

For life, the biggest aim is satisfaction

Can money bring it just a small fraction!

SMILE

Smile at others

Smile at your wife

Smile at your husband

Smile at your child

Smile at everyone

It doesn't matter who it is

And that will help you grow

In greater love for each other.

(MOTHER TERESA)

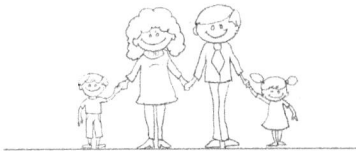

A WONDERFUL FAMILY

We have a wonderful dad

Who keeps us always glad

He gives us love and protection

And showers on us his affection

He has time to play with us

And guides us for our success

He looks like an angel of GOD

When he smiles and gives his nod

My mother is loving and caring

And brothers are always sharing

We live in our home very happily

How deeply we love our family.

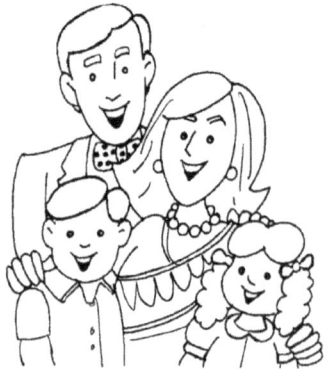

THE TRUTH

Speak the truth

Speak that is pleasant

Do not speak what is unpleasant

Do not speak what is pleasant

But untrue.

(A SANSKRIT SAYING)

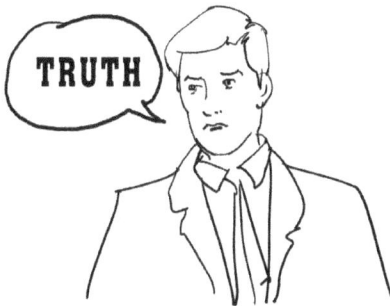

TREASURE OF KNOWLEDGE

Our knowledge

We must treasure

And use it

To help our earth

Let us boys and girls

All over the world

Unite and show our worth

This world is a family

We should live in harmony

Making our endeavours

All the while

And sharing all things

With love and smile.

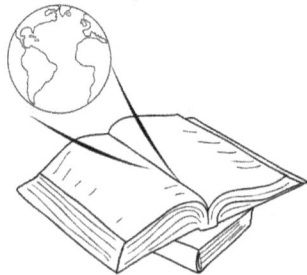

A LOVE LETTER

A love letter

Straight from your heart

Keeps us so near

Even though miles apart

I never feel alone

Either in day or at night

When I have with me

All the love you write!

THE TEST OF LIFE

Life is a test

And God at his best

In this examination

Life is an answer sheet

And we are all students

We write our answers

The time allowed is in three stages

First is the childhood

A time to play

Second is youth

To work and sway

The third and the last

We feel aghast.

When the time is over

The bell rings

And the answer sheet

Is snatched away!

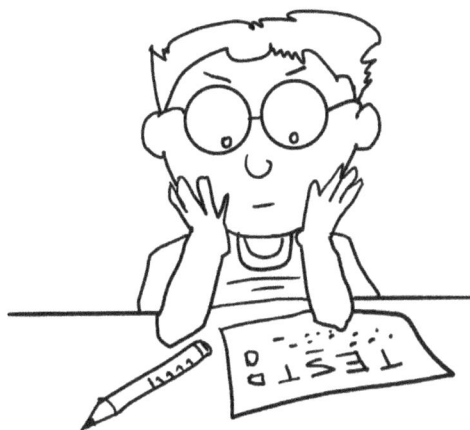

MY MOTHER

My dear mother is all affection
With love and care
God made our relation
She gave me birth
And of her love sublime
There is no dearth
She suffers whenever
Letters no word ever
Her love great and rare
God made mothers
To be everywhere!

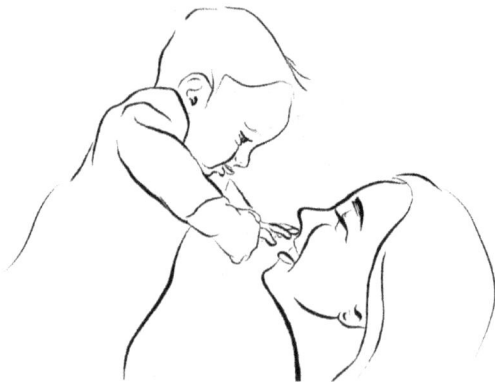

GREAT MEN

The heights achieved and kept
By great men
Were not attained in a
Sudden flight
But they while their
Companions slept
Were toiling upwards
In the night
(H.W. LONGFELLOW)

MY FRIEND

I need you my friend
Please hold my hand
In the hour of need
And give me your love
Without any greed
Love me with grace
Wipe tears from my face
And always be near
To remove doubt and fear
In this world so cold
The warmth of your touch
Will make me bold
I love you so much.

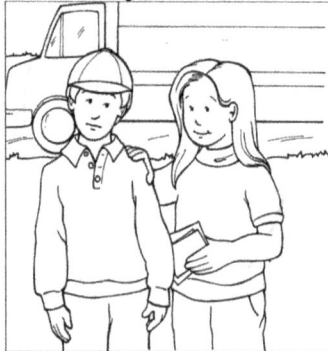

CLIMB HIGHER

Higher, higher shall we climb
Up the mount of glory
That our names may be through time
In this world's story.

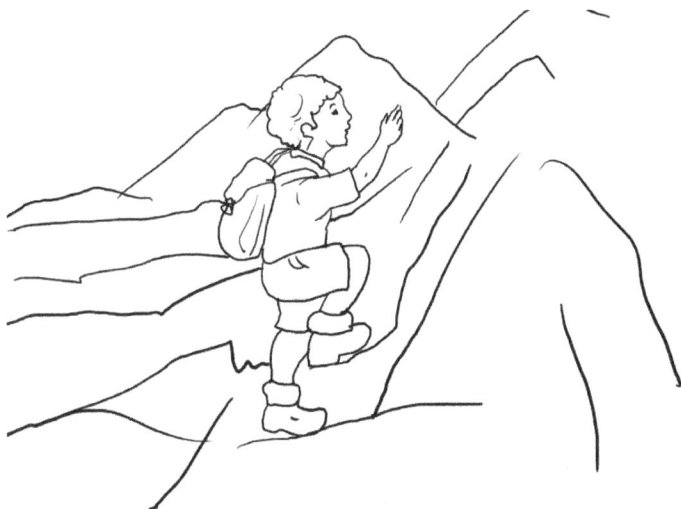

HOW SAD!

When I took birth
On this wide earth
Everyone was sad
They thought it bad
Relatives all came
To share the pain
Silent was the nurse
Said I was a curse
Become I am a girl
Stone not a pearl.
(BY A GIRL STUDENT)

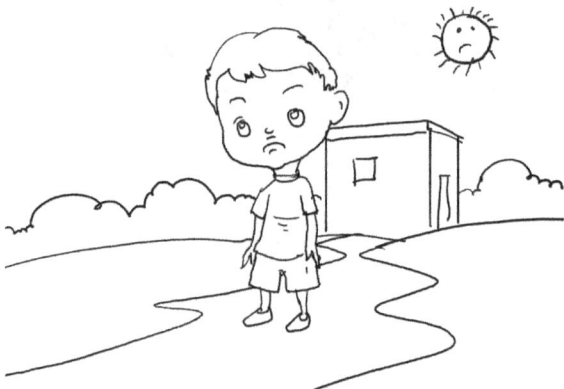

GIRLS

Girls are beautiful
Let us be thankful
Girls are so brave
Full of love and grace
KALPNA CHAWLA first woman's face
To land in space
So be kind and grateful

Girls should be treated well.
(BY A GIRL STUDENT)

A HAPPY DAY

Take one pound of kindness
And stir with thoughts of bliss
Plenty of patience makes it nice
Some fun will add a little spice
Do not weigh love pour it anyway
Mix well, you will have a HAPPY DAY!
                    (WOLFE)

A SYMPATHETIC WOMAN

Who inspires a man – a good woman!
Who interests him – a brilliant woman!
Who fascinates him – a beautiful woman!
But who really wins him
A sympathetic woman!
(ANONYMOUS)

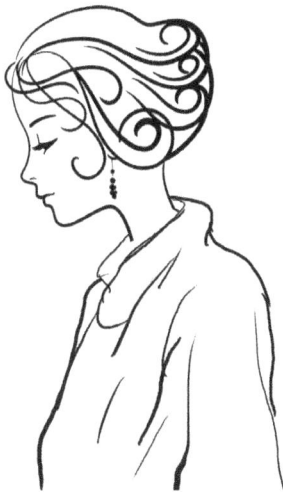

WHAT A LIFE

What life have you if you
Have not life together
There is no life that is not
In community
And no community
Not living in praise of GOD.
                    (T.S.ELIOT)

LOVE IS THE LAW OF LIFE

All love is expansion
All selfishness contraction
Love is the law of life
He who loves lives
While the selfish dies
Therefore love
For love's sake as
It is the law of life
Just as you breathe
      (SWAMI VIVEKANANDA)

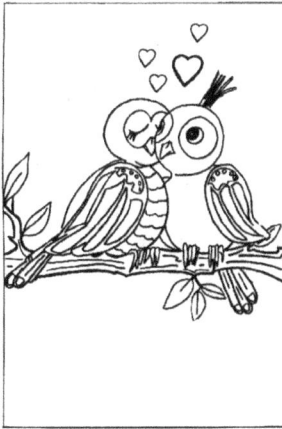

WOMAN

Adore women, Wordsworth commended her
Shakespeare loved her, Tolstoy planted her
In sunshine and watered her with tears
Burns smiled at her; Henry James studied her
De Maupassant thought she was interesting
Bourget criticized her.
BALZAC understood her
Only GOD made her!
(ANONYMOUS)

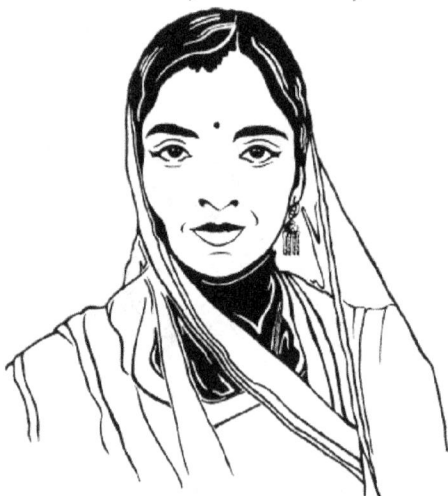

BE MY FRIEND

Do not walk behind me
I may not lead
Do not walk in front of me
I may not follow
Just walk beside me
And be my friend.
(ALBERT CAMUS)

FRIEND AND ENEMY

He who has a thousand friends
Has not a friend to spare
And he who has one enemy
Will meet him everywhere.
(ANONYMOUS)

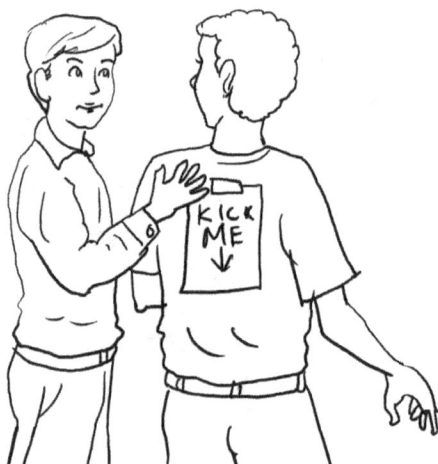

HAPPINESS

Happiness is when what you think
What you say
And what you do
Are in harmony.
(MAHATMA GANDHI)

WANTED SUCH BOYS

Boys of spirit boys of will
Boys of muscle brain and power
They are wanted every hour
Not the weak and weeping type
Who will make troubles magnify
Not they
Who may say!
I cannot do it
But the brave one who will say
I will try and I can
Whatever you do with earnest zeal
Put your shoulders to the wheel
Though your work may be hard
Do it as an honest task
In a workshop on the farm
At the desk wherever you be
From your honest efforts boys
Will shape nation's destiny!

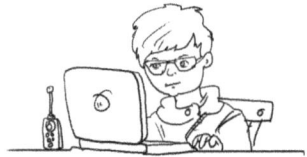

MY TEACHER AND I

If I reach classroom late
I become undisciplined
If my teacher comes late
She was too busy elsewhere
If I ask the class to stand up
When she enters the room
I am trying to act smart
If she asks the class to stand up
When the principal comes
She inculcates discipline
If I answer her questions speedily
I am trying to be clever
If she replies to the students' doubts
She is knowledgeable
If I do not do my homework
I act lazy
If she delays checking notebooks
She is checking them thorough
If I show my regard for her
I am flattering her
If she is flattering the principal
She is very cooperative.

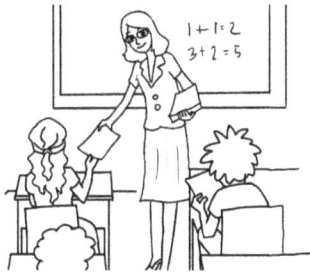

I CAN DO SOMETHING

I am only one
But I am one
I cannot do everything
But I can do something
What I can do
I ought to do
By the grace of GOD
I will do.

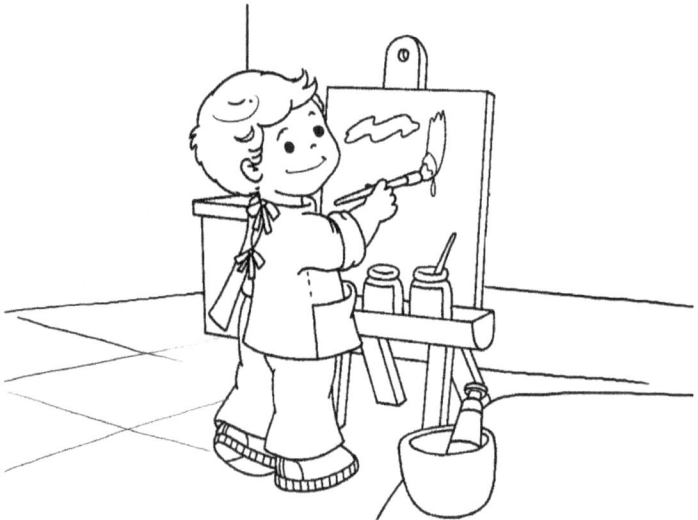

NEED AND GREED

There is enough in the world
For everyone's need
But not for one man's greed
This makes man selfish.
(KHALIL GIBRAN)

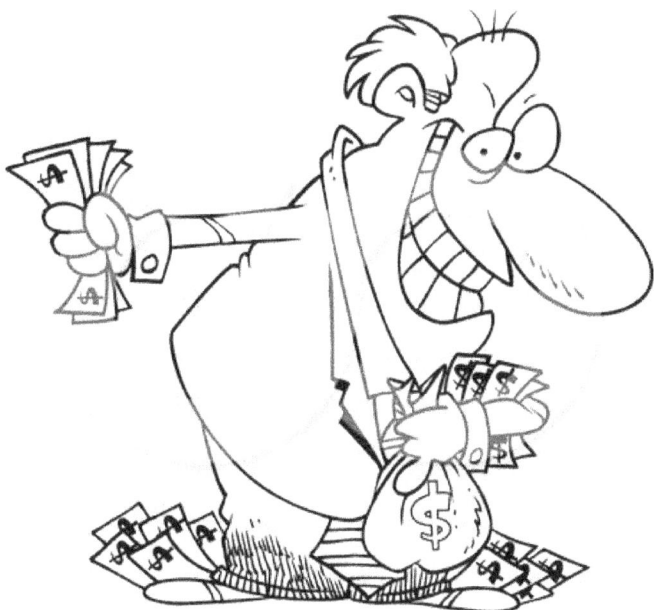

SHADES OF LIFE

Life is a boat we sail on
Life is a festival we celebrate
Life is a flower that blooms and dies
Life is of God it made us all.

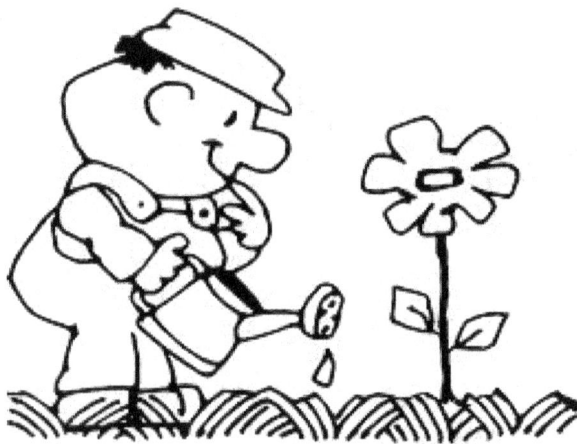

LEAD KINDLY LIGHT

Lead kindly light amid
The encircling gloom
Lead thou me on
The night is dark I am
Far from home
Lead thou me on
Keep thou my feet I do not ask to see
The distant scene one step enough for me.

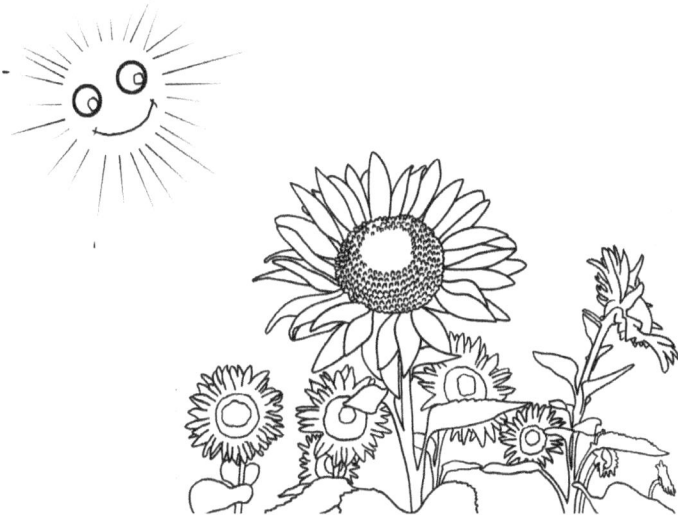

TEACHER – A CHILD'S DEAREST FRIEND

She is fine
A precious companion
A mother part time
With soothing love
She wipes away tears
With loving care
She drives away fears
Blessed with a patience rare
Gentle voice, a heart, soft and fair
A good listener, a guide worthwhile
She always wears an inspiring smile
A playmate at what a pleasant delight
A strict referee if there is a fight
She is pleasant and gay
But disciplines with firmness
If children disobey
As a companion she has much to lend
A teacher is a child's dearest friend.

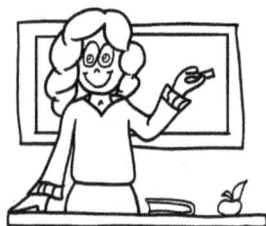

GOD OF ALL THINGS

Early in the morning
When I see
Tree tops waving
 In ghee
My heart starts singing
With joy in me!
Then I feel a presence
Of supreme delight
Which abides?
All around day and night
And all over the earth
In all the space
In every place
It is thee it is thee
Oh God of all things
My head bow in silent prayer
Come lead me and inspire
And make my life noble
With your holy light and fire.

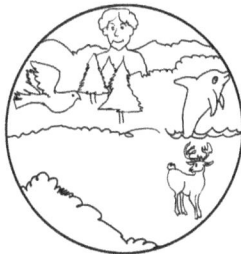

SPEECH

Speak for pleasure
Speak with measure
Speak with gentlemen treasures
Not too much
And with reflection
Deeds will follow
Word's direction.

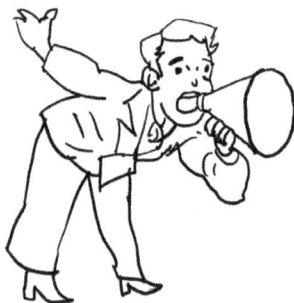

A GIRL CHILD

A girl child is a great gift to life
Mother, sister, daughter and wife
Symbols of care, love and affection
Only fools kill them!

THREE THINGS

Three things to respect – Old age, religion and law
Three things to cultivate – Cheerfulness, contentment and kindness
Three things to admire – Intellect, beauty and music
Three things to govern – Tongue, temper and taste
Three things to watch – Words, behaviour and character
Three things to love – Honesty, integrity and truth
Three things to wish – Health, happiness and prosperity
Three things to keep – Promise, friendship and affection
Three things to prevent – Laziness, falsehood and slander

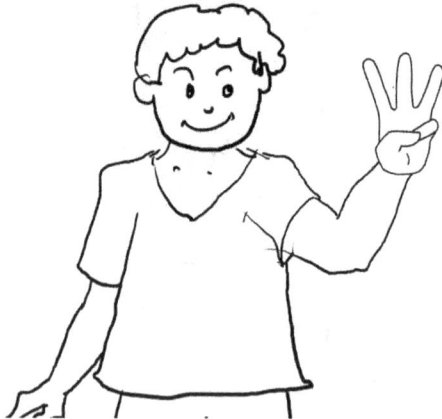

PEOPLE – GREAT AND STRONG

Not gold but only men can make
A people great and strong
Men who for truth and honour sake
Stand fast and suffer long.
                    (EMERSON)

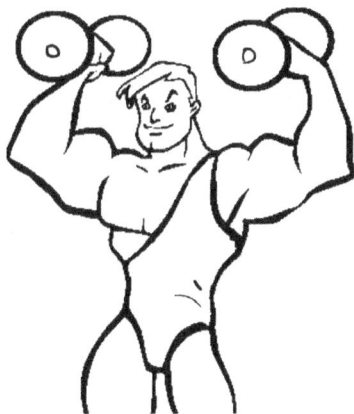

FRUITS OF EVIL DEEDS

Neither in the skies
Nor in the ocean depths
Not in the mountain caves
Nor anywhere on the earth's face
Is there a spot to lend?
Where man can escape!
The fruits of his evil deeds.

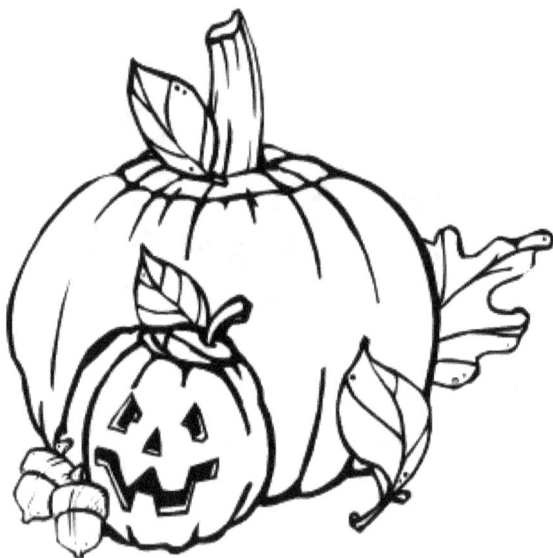

THE MAGIC OF THE MIND

There are times
When nothing seems to go right
No matter what you try
But all we utter is a cry
That is the time to fight
To know and act for victory
Both loss and gain
All pleasures and pain
Are brought by thoughts
Of different kinds
The failure
Of all thoughts
Is spam
By the magic of the mind!

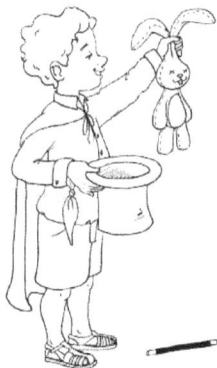

THREE CLASSES OF MAN

One who runs after money!
Is money mad!
If he hoards money
It is his fad
If he spends it all with joy
He is a playboy
If he hardly gets and keeps cool
People call him a fool
So think free before you
Amass wealth
Without caring for morals
And good health.

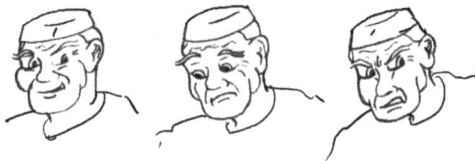

ROLE OF TIME

Time will come and slowly go
Our spirit is high and version low
Time sometimes makes us sad
It is then we feel very bad
Sometimes we may feel depressed
And sometimes we feel stressed
To be happy, spend your time
As if you are reaching a rhyme!
Be happy and laugh a while,
To enable you walk mile after mile.

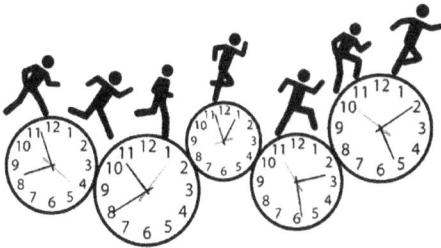

ROLE OF LOVE

All love is expansion
And selfishness contraction
Love is the law of life
In comfort or in strife
He who loves really lives
The selfish while living dies
Love for love's sake
It is the law of life to take.

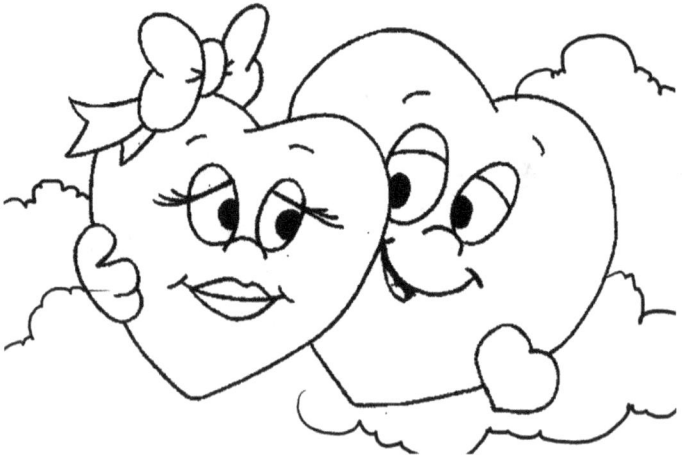

PROPER USE OF TIME

Take time to think
It is the source of power
Take time to read
It is the basis of wisdom
Take time to play
It is the secret of youth
Take time to pray
It is the source of strength
Take time to love
It is a gift of God
Take time to be friendly
It is the path of happiness
Take time to laugh
It is the music of soul
Take time to give
It is an act of service
Take time to work
It is the price of success!

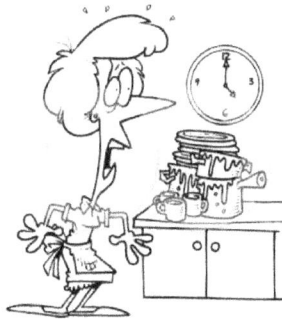

DEAR DAUGHTER

When God created daughters he took
Very special care to find
The precious treasures that would
Make them fair and kind
He made them from sugar
And a little bit of spice
He blessed them with sweet laughter
And everything that is nice
God smiled when he made daughter
Because he knew that
He had created love and joy
For every mom and father.
(COURTESY, HINDUSTAN TIMES)

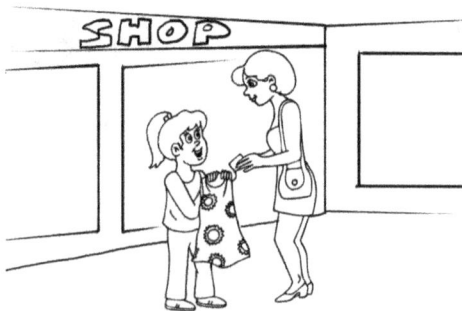

MY NAME IS TODAY

I roam in the street
With no one to greet!
And pick up all rags
Without any rich tags
And wade through filth
Barefoot and unkempt
Without a sense of guilt
You may see me at the junction
Where I have to perform
My daily life function
Of begging for money
To eat some bread
Without milk and honey
I sleep on a footpath
And fear with public wrath
Or in a dingy park
Where dogs often bark
And dream of some day
To feel happy and gay
Next day I get up again
To go to another lane
To repeat the same story.

How sad and glory
It is all dark and sorrow
For me there is no tomorrow
Every tomorrow becomes today
For me every day is today
So call me whatever you may
But my name is today
You see my every day
My name is today!
(ANONYMOUS)

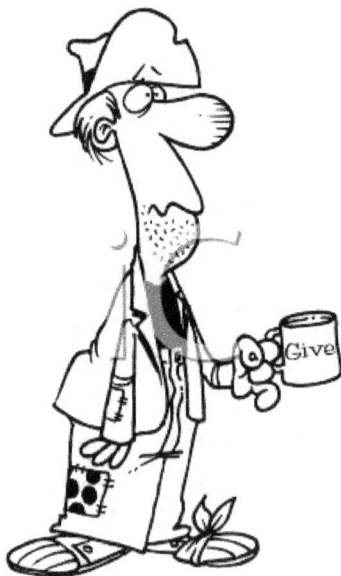

EARLY IN THE MORNING

Early in the morning
When I see
Tree tops dancing
In glee
My heart starts singing
With joy in me.
I feel a presence
Of supreme delight
Which abides all around?
Through day and night
Spread all over the earth
And in the space
In every place
It is thee it is thee
O God of all, you and me!

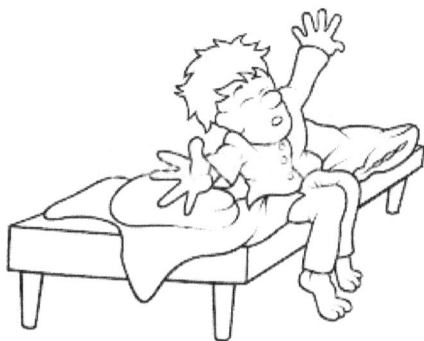

FACE OF A CHILD

How innocent is a child's face
Full of charm and divine grace
Like a flower full of light
Spreads joy and gives delight
Always engrossed doing something
Smiling and weeping washing and sleeping
Rolling on, crawling, bubbling and juggling
Playing with ease or sometimes struggling
With face lit up often with a smile
Has no prejudice, pride or guide
Friendly to all and hatred for none
He hugs with love all and one
Born as a child has grown as a man
God grant me our boon if you can
Free me from the drudgery of pleasure and pain,
And make me a little child once again.

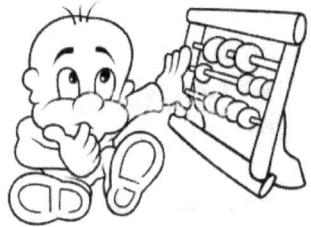

—

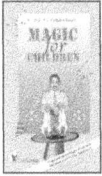

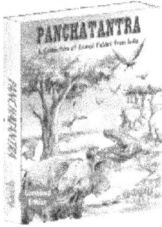

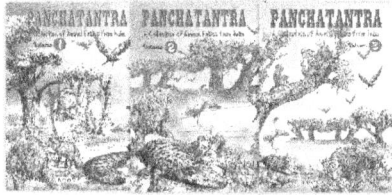

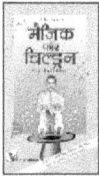

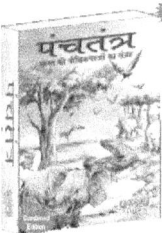

All Books Fully Coloured

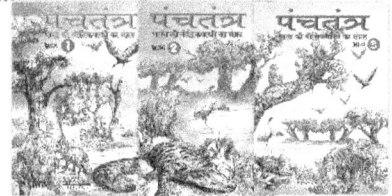

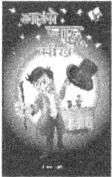

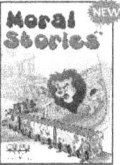

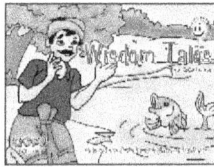

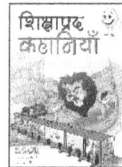

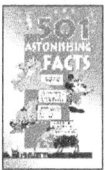

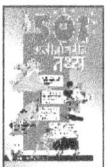

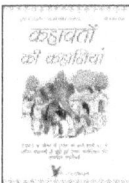

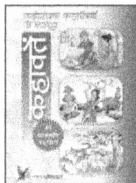

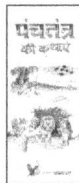

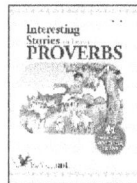

All books available at www.vspublishers.com

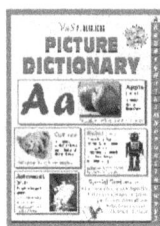

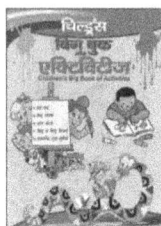

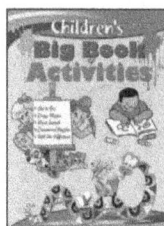

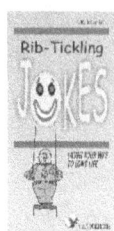

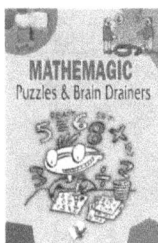

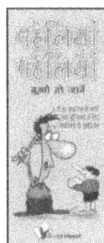

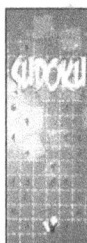

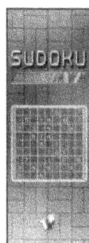

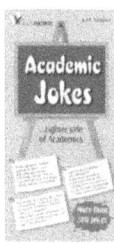

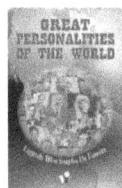

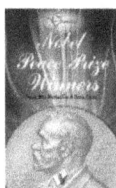

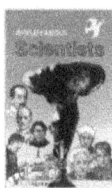

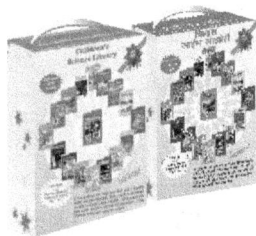

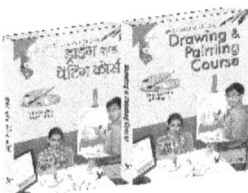

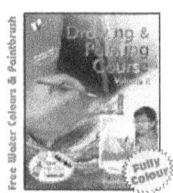

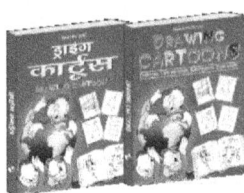

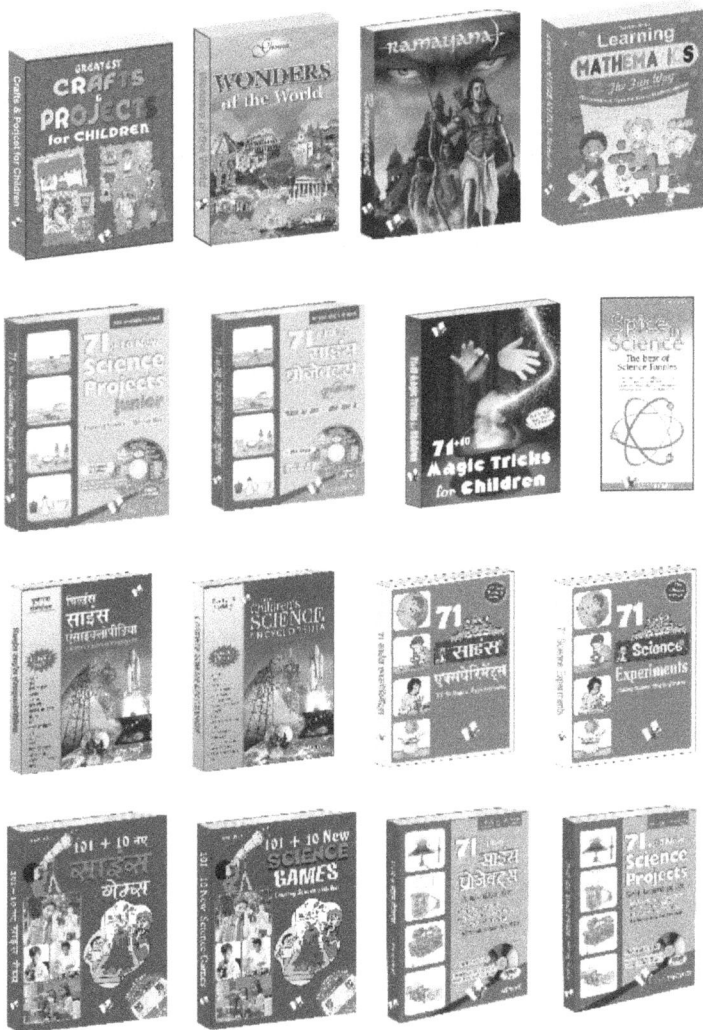